LONGEVITY WITH HEALTHY, VIBRANT ENERGY FOR LIFE!

Syncing Heart Intelligence, Brain Willpower and Divine Self.

JUNE SCHAMP, BSC, BHS

Balboa Press books may be ordered through booksellers or by contacting:

Balboa Press
A Division of Hay House
1663 Liberty Drive
Bloomington, IN 47403
www.balboapress.com
1 (877) 407-4847

ISBN: 978-1-9822-4117-9 (sc)
ISBN: 978-1-9822-4118-6 (e)

Library of Congress Control Number: 2020931541

Print information available on the last page.

Balboa Press rev. date: 02/28/2020

BALBOA.PRESS

As a portal of love, light, and healing, to my children,

Dale, Debbie, Wendy, and Wayne;

to my grandchildren,

Brandon, Sheridan, Heather, and Sydney

to my sister,

Joy,

who listens patiently to my endless musings;

to Carroll,

my partner, companion, and husband;

To every child of the universe

who is "hanging out" in a human body here on planet Earth;

and to my mum and dad,

*who are no longer on Earth but, while here, gave me an abundance of everything
I needed to get started on my adventure as a human being on planet Earth.*

Much love and gratitude!

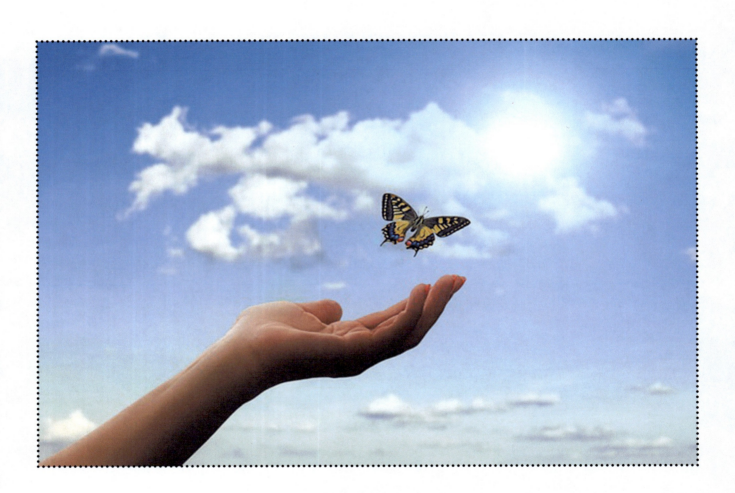

Introduction

My name is June Schamp, and I am a subtle-energy healer. I am aware of how stress is affecting our lives in our rapidly changing, busy world. Stress is held in our muscles as tension and in our joints as pain and stiffness. It diminishes our energy flow, and our overwhelmed brains are unable to respond to life's challenges and precious moments intelligently. What can we do to regain an abundance of healthy, vibrant energy for life?

I graduated with a BSc in healing science from the prestigious Barbara Brennan School of Healing in 2007 and then passionately pursued a wide spectrum of other natural healing modalities—from quantum levels of energy healing to healing aspects of diet, exercise, and hydration. I also discovered that what we believe, what we think about, and our level of conscious awareness also affect the level of health in our bodies and minds.

As I attended workshops and collected information and certifications from some of the most respected healers, scientists, and mentors in the world, a nagging question was always in my awareness: Can our bodies and minds really heal themselves?

With great confidence, I can now say, "Yes, they can."

Is it easy to do? Not for most people. However, if you sincerely desire to have an abundance of healthy, vibrant energy for life and are willing to live your life a bit differently, I can show you information, along with revolutionary tools, tips, and routines to help you experience the miracles of being well and enjoying longevity that is rich in self-determination.

Becoming well can be achieved by developing different attitudes and routines that allow you to enjoy the freedom to direct your own destiny and maintain longevity of ideas. You can do this with clear emotional mental abilities as well as exceptional physical health and live life to its fullest at any age with passion, understanding, and a feeling of fulfillment.

As human beings, we live with other life forms on a beautiful living planet called Earth. We all have various degrees of consciousness. Plant, mineral, and animal kingdoms live with us on planet Earth in the natural process of life. There has to be death to make space for the new. Human beings have the capacity to reverse that entropy, that degeneration or breaking down, because we are conscious beings.

We have consciousness. Plants, animals, and minerals also have a level of consciousness but are not conscious of the fact that they are living toward or moving toward dying. Animals do not think about it; they don't think, *Oh, I am born, and now I am living to die.* Nor do plants and minerals. They are not aware that it is going to happen in their reality. Human beings, on the other hand, are aware of this process, and we can be worried about it or scared of it. But because we are conscious beings, we are also capable of slowing and reversing that process through consciousness and doing so begins with diet and exercise.

Going beyond the physical body, we recognize that we also have mental and emotional bodies and etheric or energy bodies, which current research and science now agree exist. Our physical bodies spring forth from a pure well of divine source energy. Some folks speak of this energy as God/Goddess/All That Is energy. All is ultimately energy and the shapes and forms our thoughts spin create their own vibration or frequency. Everything has its own unique frequency. Later in this book, we will examine this more closely. We will see how these frequencies of vibration can become damaged or blocked and affect our states of being well.

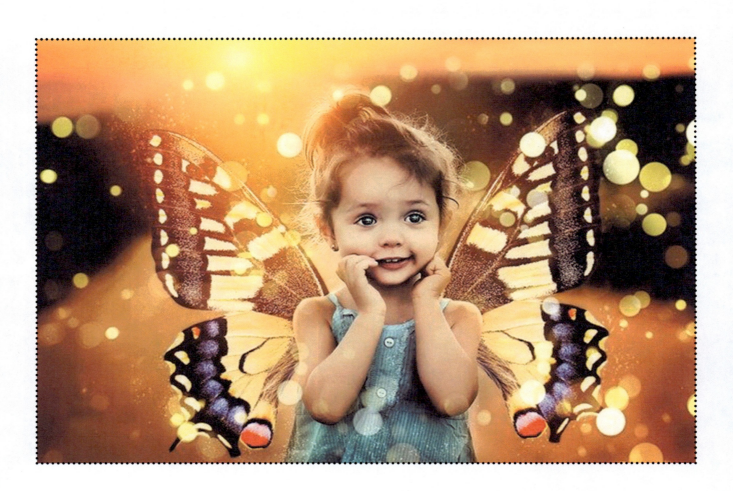

Part I

CREATING YOUR MAP

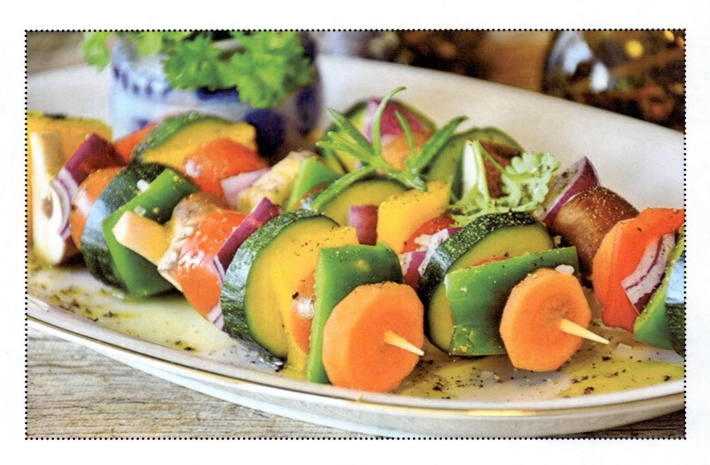

Diet

Chapter 1

Diet

I begin in this first part with the physical body and focus here on diet, exercise, dominion with nature, and the importance of work and play.

At this level, we can begin to reverse entropy, the deteriorating or breaking-down process that can be a natural process in life. If not worked with consciously, this process can lead to disease and an early death. Our bodies and minds have no desire to deteriorate, grow weak, or die earlier than what is right for each of us.

When it comes to *diet*, many of us go online and try to locate the best diets. Well, they can all work, and none of them can work. Diet is an individual thing, so listen to your body. It will let you know which one is best for you. Experiment. You may choose a diet with some meat, no meat, gluten, no gluten, vegan only—or maybe not. Over time, as you become more aware of subtle messages from your body and mind, you will clearly see which diet is best for you. Listed below are some things to remember when enjoying your food:

TOP 5 REASONS TO BUY ORGANIC FOODS TODAY

1. Avoid harmful chemicals

Eating organically grown foods is the only way to avoid the cocktail of chemical poisons present in commercially grown food.

2. Benefit from more nutrients

Organically grown foods have more nutrients—vitamins, minerals, enzymes, and micronutrients—than commercially grown foods because the soil is managed and nourished with sustainable practices by responsible standards.

3. Enjoy better taste

Try it! Organically grown foods generally taste better because nourished, well balanced soil produces healthy, strong plants.

4. Avoid GMO

Genetically engineered (GE) food and genetically modified organisms (GMO) are contaminating our food supply at an alarming rate, with repercussions beyond understanding. GMO foods do not have to be labeled in America.

5. Avoid hormones, antibiotics and drugs in animal products

Conventional meat and dairy are the highest risk foods for contamination by harmful substances. More than 90% of the pesticides Americans consume are found in the fat and tissue of meat and dairy products.

Eat small portions five to six times per day. The stomach is the size of a fist, so going without food and then eating a large meal later in the day is not good for the well-being of your body and mind. It can upset your digestive system and actually give you a headache and interrupt your sleep.

Eat fresh, organically grown fruits and vegetables when you can.

- Eat locally grown produce and foods when you can. However, be aware of what you are buying. Sometimes, flash frozen produce can retain more healthy nutrients than fresh, organic, locally grown produce that has been sitting out on the farmer's market table for a day or so and has become wilted and dehydrated. Flash frozen food items have been frozen quickly at extremely low temperatures with cold circulating air. This process allows food items to retain more nutrients and juices than if you purchase them at the grocery store and then placed them in your freezer at home.

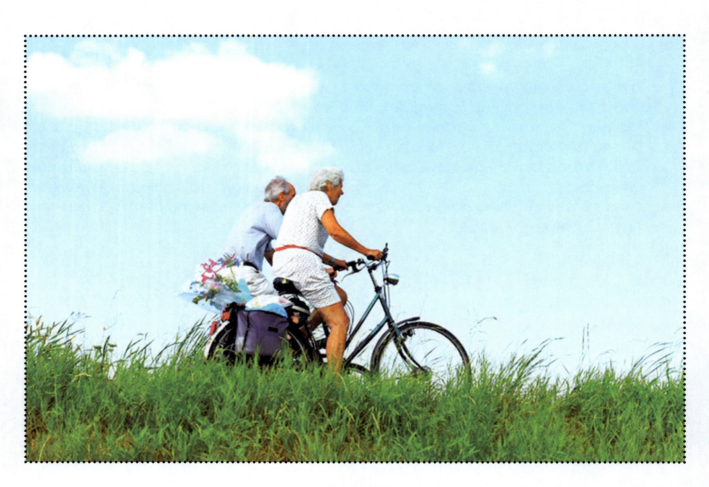

Exercise

Chapter 2

Exercise

Exercise is critical in reversing the process of entropy. Some people love exercise, and others resist it. However, just know that you need to exercise a minimum of two times per week. Three times is better, and four or more is best if you enjoy exercise. Create a routine with at least two exercise sessions of twenty to thirty minutes each week and do it every week. Walk, go to the gym, or participate in a sport. The plan is to stimulate blood flow beyond your normal rate.

Listed below are some things to remember when exercising:

- Always cool down; it is very important. It's not good to just stop and have the blood slam up against your arteries.

- Drink plenty of clean water regularly. (The importance of staying hydrated will be discussed later.)

TOP 5 IMPORTANT REASONS TO EXERCISE

1. Weight Control

One of the most common benefits of exercise is that it helps you control and manage your weight. Exercise burns calories, which results in shedding pounds.

2. Physical Fitness

Exercise doesn't just keep you trim—it helps you stay healthy. Regular exercise increases your overall level of fitness, which in turn boosts your immune system and makes you more resilient to illnesses like the common cold.

3. Energy

One of the reasons to exercise regularly is that it gives you energy. A workout can help oxygen flow more freely throughout the body and give you a much-needed burst of energy to get you through the day. It also increases your overall stamina and sense of wellbeing.

4. Mental Health

Exercise has been proven to provide a mood booster, as it releases chemicals into your brain that help you feel happier and can ease the effects of depression, ADHD, and anxiety. It can also allow you to sleep better at night,

5. Long-term Health

Regular exercise can help prevent heart disease and diabetes in the long term. Working out increases your "good" cholesterol and can help with a myriad of health issues. Begin with taking a simple walk. Try to work physical activity into your daily routine one step at a time.

- Make sure you add a stretching routine into your exercise routine. Yoga is excellent. Hold the stretch firm and do not bounce. You can integrate stretching exercises into your warm-up practice. Just stretch. It releases lactic acid from your muscles, allows joints to stay flexible, and releases the aches, stiffness, and pain that quickly build up when stretching exercises are neglected.

- It is also important to practice a balancing exercise with your stretching routine. Stand on one leg supported by your hand on a chair or wall for a few moments every day, and then reverse by standing on the other leg. This short exercise is critical in maintaining a sense of inner stamina and balance.

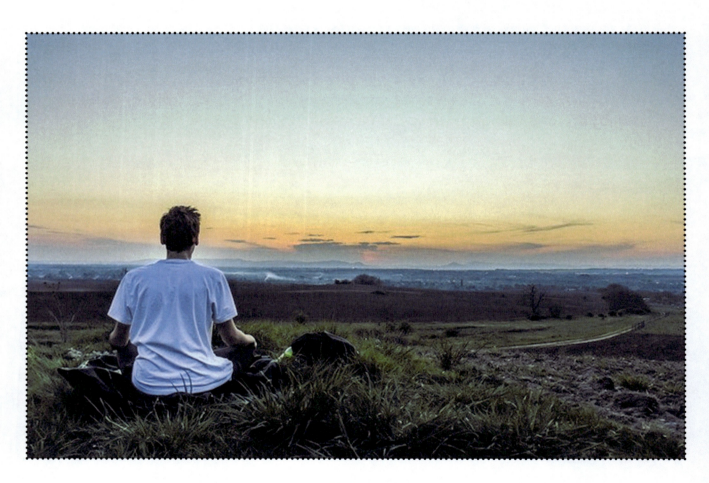

Nature

Chapter 3

Dominion with Nature

Basically, this means be with nature. Walk in nature. Honor nature. With planning, this step can be integrated into your exercise routine, or you can make time and space in your life for connection with source energy through nature. This time is important in reversing the process of entropy.

Be aware of the four elements; they are present all around and within you. They are essential to all life. You and the universe are formed by these four elements—earth, air, water, and fire. These elements go beyond the physical and manifest as personality traits and energetic forces too. The elements are here to bring balance. Fire needs water to be quenched, and the earth needs wind to move it. Being with the elements brings balance to your personality.

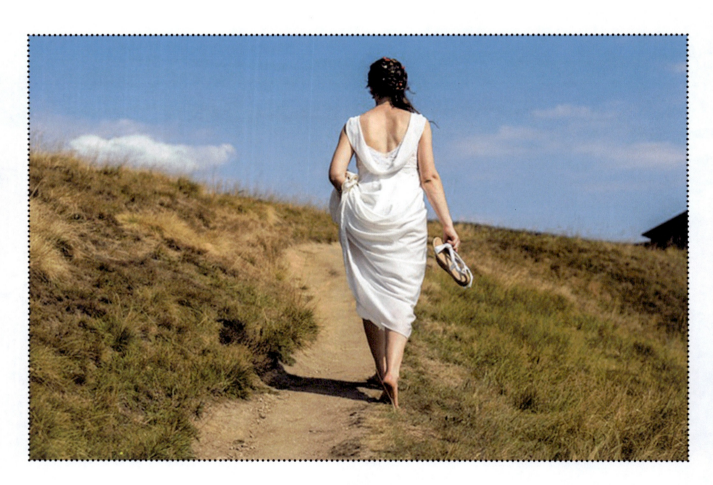

Grounding

Listed are some ideas of how to connect with the four elements:

- *Earth element*—Walk barefoot when you can. The routines of exercise and diet are connected to the earth element. Commit to your routines. Sleep patterns are also connected with the earth element, so develop a routine for going to bed at night and for getting up in the morning. Become aware of how many hours of sleep you need and try to conform to a routine. Do the best you can but do plan at least six hours each night. Earthing products are now available and can be found online. They are basically "extension cords" that bring Earth's energy from outside into the inside of your office or home—simulating being barefoot outside. These products are in the form of sheets and pads and address the issue of comfort, convenience, and reality. They are helpful, especially if you are sleeping in a room that is several stories off the ground, as in high-rise buildings.

- *Air element*—Take time to practice conscious breathing. Practice diaphragmatic breathing, alternate nostril breathing, or heart breathing. Basically, consciously inhale slowly and a little more deeply for five seconds and out for five seconds in sets of three. Practice several times per day or as needed.

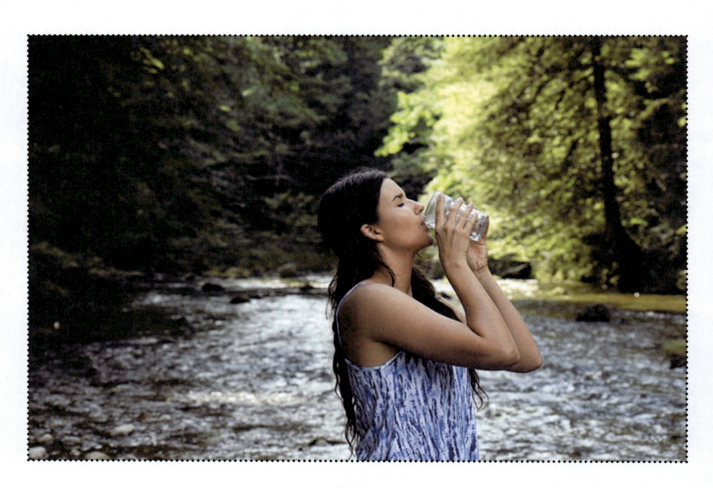

Water

- *Water element*—Drink water. Your body needs water. Take baths. Spend at least ten minutes in the shower or twenty minutes in the tub every day. Your skin will absorb the water and become more hydrated. You need internal cellular hydration, as well as external hydration. Splash your face with water several times every day. It will reverse entropy of your skin. Your hands absorb a lot of energy; wash them often to keep them hydrated. Remember to keep your hands away from your nose, mouth, and eyes as much as you can, because your hands come in contact with many energies that you do not want to enter your body.

- *Fire element*—Our bodies need the element of fire, and it comes to us in the sun's rays. Our bodies need sunlight. They need to absorb some UVB rays, which are part of UV rays, and we need to absorb the rays through our bare skin. The best way to do this is to spend ten minutes early in the morning and ten minutes in the late afternoon. It is important to *not* wear sunblock or sunglasses during this time. I remind you that I am not saying to spend an excess amount of time baking in the sun. If you must spend excess time out in the sun, then use sunblock and sunglasses, but do not expose any area of your body to the sun for more than twenty minutes. The sun also provides us with nutrients, warmth, and healing energy. It provides a balancing effect on and in our bodies when used appropriately.

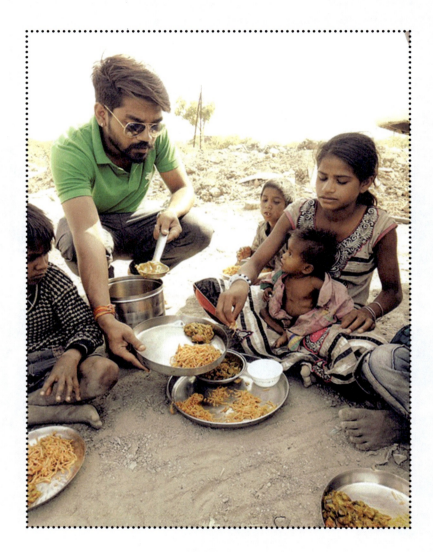

Work

Chapter 4

Work

Continue to work throughout your life because it is very important and very critical to longevity. It can be work with no payment, as in volunteer work, or it can be work for payment. Work needs to continue throughout the fullness of life. It's essential. It's part of reversing entropy. If you don't have the energy of work integrated in your life, there is room for entropy to start destroying the cellular structure and the mental structure.

Energetically, in between work and play, certain energies need to be present in our lives:

To be of service. Be of service to others in some way, perhaps through your *play* or through your *work*.

Two energies best present in our work are *intimacy* and *caring*. Be close, be tender, and be vulnerable and trusting with your coworkers and with your company's policies. And adopt an attitude of cooperation within your working schedule. Also, within your working relationships, do care and love at the level of understanding. Embellish your work with these qualities. Be caring in your work. It will become rewarding and fulfilling in this way.

TOP 5 REASONS TO WORK/PLAY THROUGHOUT YOUR LIFE

1. Happiness

Healthy, happy people have a diversity of experience and are able to cycle in and out of work and play. Being "out of the game" means you are no longer seen as a player and with that comes a loss of friends and events that you previously enjoyed.

2. Health

Maintaining a working schedule of paid work or non-paid work is a healthy think to do. It helps maintain some structure in one's life and usually requires some degree of continued learning which helps maintain mental clarity.

3. Relationships

Traditional retirement often brings about a change in relationships and quite frequently puts added stress on a marriage. Diversity in lifestyle creates more coherent communications and joyful moments with those that matter to you.

4. Finances

Accepting payment for work and for many people there is a need for additional income.

5. Wellbeing

Creating a life filled with family, fitness, leisure, travel education and work in an everchanging mix leads one feeling a sense of fulfillment and wellbeing.

There are also two energies tied into *play*, and they support the creative foundation of play. One of those energies is *wisdom*, and it's something that the child and adolescent lack. Wisdom can make play so much more powerful, so much more important, and so much more magical for the adult than it could ever be for the child and adolescent in this regard. The other energy to engage with play is *passion*. Awaken the energies of passion in your play. Feel joy in your play.

It is also important to allow caring and passion to be present in and critical to service. Physical, emotional, and mental energies come in here to support the foundation of healing that is built from the love and caring you feel. Then balance is built within passion and wisdom. And this leads to a greater love and a greater healing that holds and lifts you into fulfillment, which is rich in the energies of mystery and mastery that create the foundation of fulfillment.

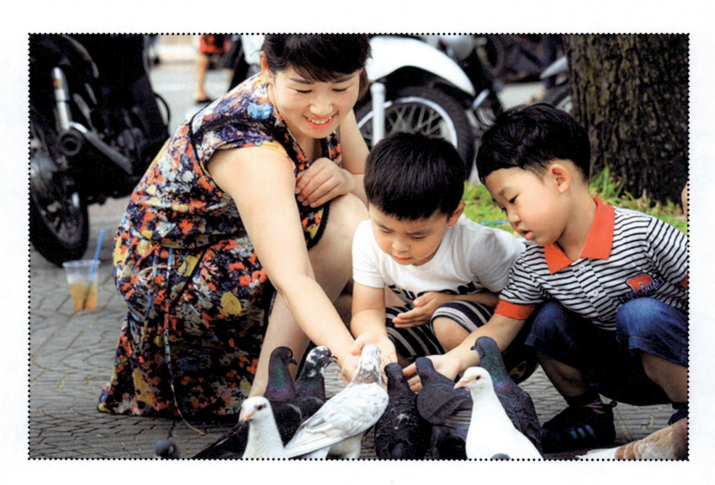

Play

Chapter 5

Play

Play is very important. Do not leave it out of your life. Do not underestimate its importance, because it is also critical in reversing entropy. Play becomes much more important as you mature and grow older.

Recreation is to engage the desire to create and engage the energies of childhood. As an adult, you can know and have the wisdom of play in a way that no child or adolescent could begin to understand, and you can also have the bounty and benefit of play that no child or adolescent has ever experienced. So be creative and play. Make your life rich with play and feel your vitality and an abundance of energy available to you every day.

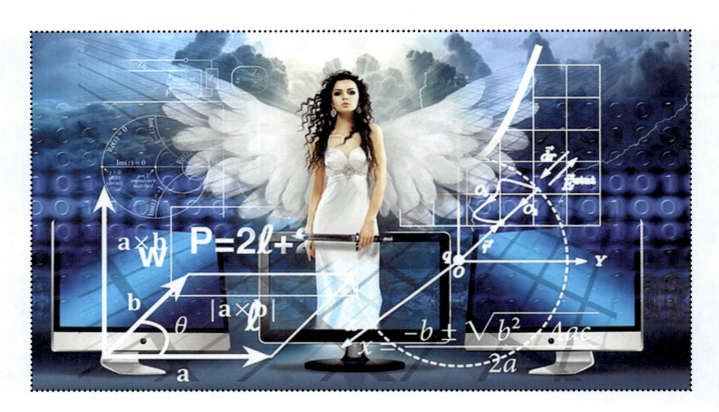

Technology

Part II

MIRACLES OF SCIENCE, TECHNOLOGIES, AND INTUITION

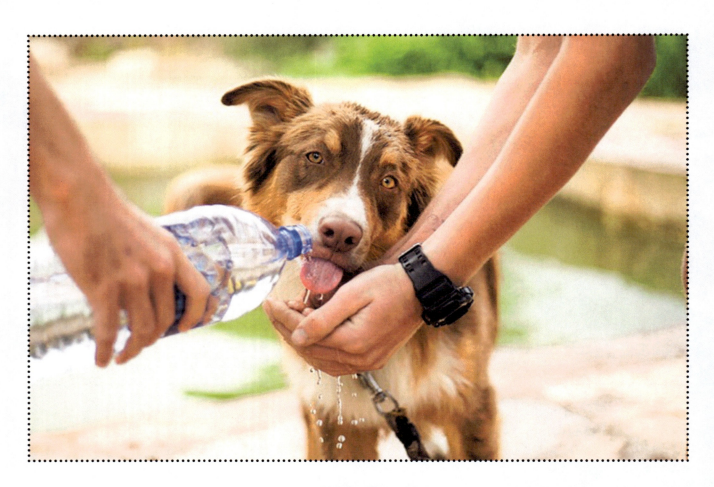

Hydration

Chapter 6

Importance of Water and Hydration

In Part I, a map or guide was developed to give you a basic, mostly physical outline of what you need to do to begin your journey to *Longevity with Healthy, Vibrant Energy for Life*. You have learned how to create a healthy diet that is right for you and how to develop an exercise routine that you can stick to and have become aware of how critical it is to continue to work and play throughout your entire life—to prevent and reverse entropy. Additionally, you learned how essential it is to be involved in some form of service to others and also to imprint positive attitudes in your mind as you go about your daily routines. This is how you begin. This is the front line to begin to reverse entropy.

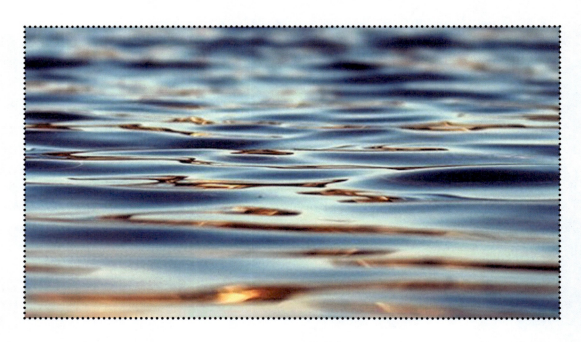

Divine Water

In this part, I will offer you information and assistance using revolutionary technologies, science, and tools and techniques to engage your heart's intuition. Intuition is the highest form of intelligence. For centuries there have been extraordinary people who have engaged their intuition and brought helpful wisdom to others in various unique ways—easing the suffering human beings often experience while living their lives. Now we are in a time when technology and your intuitive intelligence are working together. New revolutionary products using advanced technologies are available that can help you engage with and anchor in a strong, inner trust of your intuition—a sacred, inner space that is perfect for the reversal of entropy. I'll begin by sharing my exciting experiences with water and hydration.

Water

In 2006, my life was profoundly transformed when I attended a workshop with Dr. Masaro Emoto, author of *The Hidden Messages in Water*. During the following year, I attended more workshops and received more training with Dr. Emoto and ultimately received certification from him. As a certified Hado instructor, personally trained by Dr. Emoto, I am fully prepared to share Dr. Emoto's teachings and am honored to be a person who resonates with *hado* (the Japanese word for energy). According to ancient Chinese medicine and philosophy, everything releases energy or chi. In the Japanese spiritual community, Hado is a similar life-force energy that encompasses healing properties and transformative powers and is a novel philosophy that can harmonize all things. Hado is the principle of peace, represented by Dr. Emoto's water crystal images.

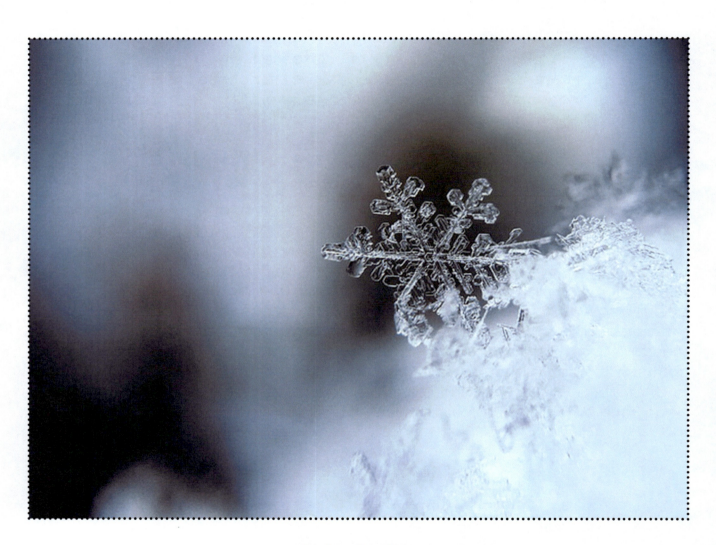

Water Crystals

The implications of his research created a new awareness of how we can positively impact the earth and our personal health. Dr. Emoto studied the scientific evidence of how the molecular structure in water transforms when it is exposed to human words, thoughts, sounds and intentions. The average human body is 70 percent water. We start out in life being 99 percent water, as fetuses. At the time of our birth, we are 90 percent water and by the time we reach adulthood, we are down to 70 percent. If we die of old age, we will probably be about 50 percent water. In other words, throughout our lives *we exist mostly as water.*

From a physical perspective, humans are water. When I realized this and started to look at the world from this perspective, I began to see things in a whole new way. The first thing I became aware of was that this connection to water applies to everyone and all life on our planet. So, I asked myself once again, with this new awareness, the question: How can people live long, happy and healthy lives?

My intuition spoke clearly of the need for all life to create an internal and external environment with clean, healthy water that makes up 70 percent of our body. This is not an easy task, with the toxic environment present everywhere on our planet these days. The water must remain clean.

Water in a river remains pure because it's moving. When water becomes trapped, it dies. Therefore, water must constantly be circulating. An article I found interesting stated that the water or blood in the bodies of the sick is usually stagnant. When blood stops flowing, the body starts to decay. Water serves as the transporter of energy throughout the body.

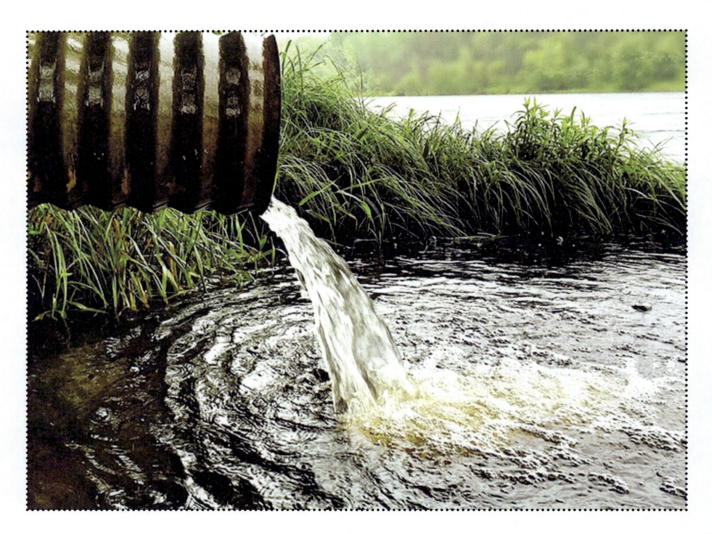

Nature's Water

Dr. Emoto's research shows water has the ability to *copy* and *memorize* information. Research has shown that water is sensitive to the unique frequencies being emitted by the outside world; it essentially and efficiently mirrors the outside world.

Amazingly, in 2016, I connected with another extraordinary man by the name of Clayton Nolte, who was also aware of Dr. Emoto's work and aware of the magical properties of water—clean, pure water. Clayton had a vision. He had spent the last forty years of his life exploring physics, math, and the properties of water and the effects it has on life. He delved into the inner world of water. Clayton is a researcher and inspired inventor of life-transforming water structuring technologies. His mission is to provide structured water to every man, woman, and child on the face of this earth in his lifetime. I share in his mission. More information about Clayton's water structuring devices can be seen at www.divinewatershop.com.

What is structured water?

Most simply put, structured water is water that has been returned to its original state through nature's natural movement. As Clayton explains, "If we take a bucket of tap water and drop it into the top of a mountain stream and then if we were able to collect that same water at the bottom of the stream after it has passed through all the twists and turns at break-neck speed, we would have a bucket of *Structured Water*." It is the vortex motion—the water swirling around rocks, churning left and right—as it rushes downward that changes its molecular structure at the hydrogen bond angle.

TOP 5 REASONS TO DRINK STRUCTURED WATER

1. Quality

When tap water passes over a particular geometric shape like the ones in the Structured Water Units, it then begins a vortex type spin state which allows the water to become structured. It is the same phenomenon that occurs when water runs down a river and hits boulders and rocks.

2. Detoxes

It is this movement of water, in the vortex energy, that changes the molecular structure of water, breaking up the memory of all it has passed through, bringing harmony to everything in its path. This is the way water moves in nature and creates pure water. Neutralizes toxins.

3. Hydration

Dehydration is the root cause of many diseases associated with aging (e.g. arthritis, GI disorders, and senile dementia). Structured water holds excess stable oxygen and is able to deliver this oxygen to cells to a greater degree than ordinary water. Real hydration gives you a better brain, a better body, a better day and a better future.

4. Benefits

Tastes delicious, water is alive and full of energy, more moisture for skin and hair, greater sense of wellbeing, no hard water build-up in shower, anti-aging, improves health, less joint and muscle pain.

5. Structured Water Technology

Portable units, garden units, shower units, under sink units, whole house units and units for commercial use.

If you were to observe a water molecule under a high-powered microscope, you would see the angle of the bond between the oxygen and hydrogen atoms is ninety degrees. When water is structured, that bond is increased up to 180 degrees.

Dear readers, please pause and think about the following words you are about to read. What is significant about that is that this increased angle does not allow for anything of a negative vibration to attach to the water molecule. That means no viruses, no harmful bacteria, no fungi, no molds, no parasites, no hydrocarbons, no pathogens of any kind, and no electromagnetic frequencies. In short, the increased hydrogen bond refuses entry to any enemy of the water molecule's integrity.

On the flip side, it allows all vibrations of a higher beneficial frequency to ride on the water molecule. The structured water molecule acts as the carrier for everything that is life and light-enhancing. *Wow!*

Dear readers, if this sounds profound, that's because it is profound. Structured water is a gift that just keeps on giving. The benefits are too many to mention here in this limited space. To name a few, structured water:

- Ensures increased oxygen intake—more resilient immune system. Improved nutrient absorption

- Softer, healthier, skin and hair, smoother water

- Reduces harmful toxins and free radicals

- Increased energy and clarity, improved circulation

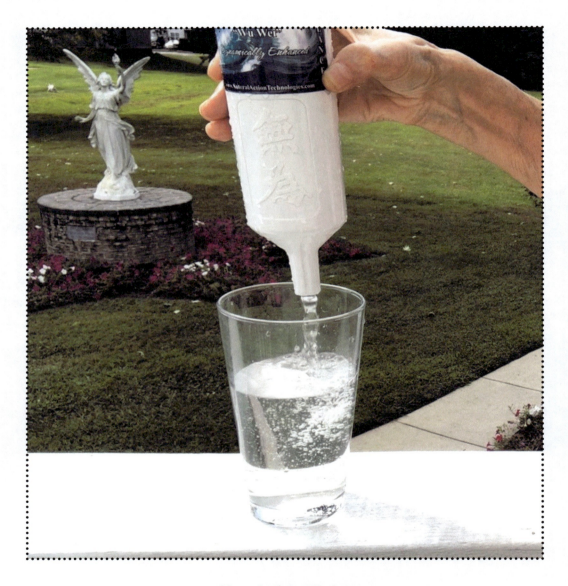

Structuring Water

Structured water also benefits animals, agriculture, and plant health. Structured water units needs no filters, no maintenance and no electricity. Portable units are the most popular, as they go everywhere with you. The whole house units make structured water instantly available for personal use and to wash or soak fruits and vegetables for eating and cooking and for all daily water use for home and garden.

Structured water is available now for you to transform the health and wellness of your family, your pets, and your gardening endeavors. For more information, go to www.divinewatershop.com. Scroll down to view products and watch the informative videos.

Water, I love you. Water, I thank you. Water, I respect you.

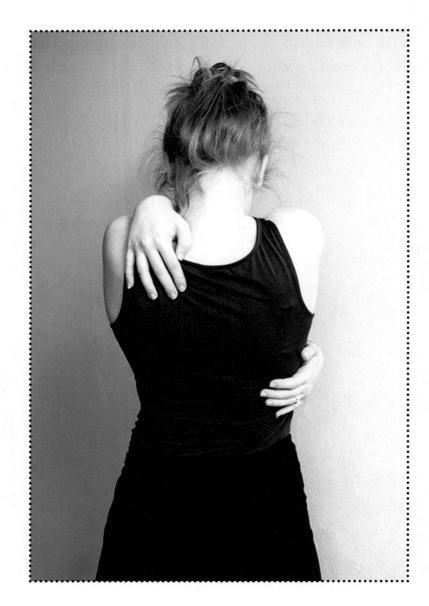

Sad

Chapter 7

Importance of Finding the Root Cause of Our Suffering

My own experiences using medicines to help me feel better have proven fruitless. Because I am a sensitive person, the side effects of the medicines caused me to suffer equal to or more than the original illness or injury. At an earlier time in my life, I spent over a week in the hospital due to a reaction to a drug prescribed for cystitis. It was dreadful, going through the tests, becoming weaker and weaker, and feeling very sick. I was frightened and thought I might die.

From that point on, I began to explore the healing delights of nature and the knowledge practiced by the ancients since the beginning of time. I became aware that everything is energy and that all matter vibrates unique frequencies of energy. And I felt there must be a way to create good health more easily, more effectively, and with a more enlightening effect.

FEATURED 5 TESTIMONIALS

1. No Further Pain—Barb B., Dover DE

No inflammation since September. I do think the water thingy is part of it. I do not use it 100% of the time but use it a lot. I often take a huge bottle of it with me to work and pour from the bottle into a glass some of the structured water and drink. I keep the device at home. Grateful for no more pain.

"(Water thingy" is NES Structured Water Portable Unit)

2. Manages Stress-- Linda F., Hartly, DE

June is one of the most intuitive people I have ever met.

I am so happy to have the tools that June has taught me and can now manage my stress and be a more positive human being than I was before. Thanks to June and the HeartMath Building Personal Resilience Program. It works!

3. Life Changing—Sharon B., Dover, DE

I decided to embark on my very own voyage to my heart intelligence. With June at the helm as my captain I navigated my way through the program learning science backed information, techniques and tools that did indeed reduce stress. I now use the tools every day. This wonderful Voyage to Heart Intelligence Program has been truly a life changing experience for me.

4. Chronic Pain Diminished—Lynne B., Wimauma, FL

I have used my NES energy-field scanner once per month for three months and have been drinking the infoceuticals in water as recommended. I am happy to share that my chronic pain has diminished.

5. Blood Sugar Drops--D.M. Towey, Delanco, NJ

I believe my health has improved greatly since using NES Health infoceuticals. Recent blood work showed my blood glucose levels dropped 12 points in 6 months. I believe the infoceuticals were a contributing factor and plan to move forward in improving my health by continuing with the infoceuticals. I also have more energy.

The problem is that modern medicine limits itself by focusing only on trying to correct the biology and biochemistry of body and the uncomfortable symptoms of entropy. They do *nothing* about the third and most important force in your body, which is your body's bioenergy field—the very source of your health and vitality. It holds the template for all that you are. And as a result of ignorance of the importance of the body's bioenergetics, many people do not get long-term healing solutions they need.

I wanted to know what causes the cells, the biology, and biochemistry in the body to break down. I spent many years developing a heightened sense of perception (also known as high-sense perception or HSP) while attending the Barbara Brennan School of Healing. By the time I graduated, I could feel energy field blockages, sense energy field changes, and sometimes see vibrant colors around my client's body. I could also hear vibrational sound changes in my ears while working with a client. I learned to use my energy hands to clear, charge, and restructure various layers of my client's energy field and to use my voice and gentle language to soothe a person's mind.

When listening to my client's positive testimonials, I always experience a ripple of light and laughter spiral through me. It feels magical and I feel fortunate and blessed to be able to help people feel better.

As the number of clients in my energy healing practice increased, I found myself experiencing difficulties expressing clearly what I could offer my potential clients for the energy healing session fee they would be paying. I always felt I was offering them something that was invisible. I struggled with that for many, many years and always found myself searching for a better way to show my client their energy field was real.

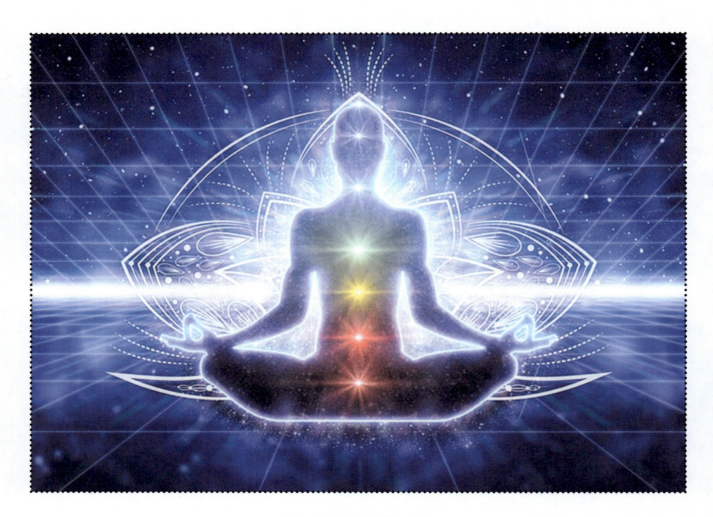

Body Energy-fields

And then it happened, I saw an article about *The Living Matrix: A Film on the New Science of Healing* displayed on my Facebook newsfeed. I experienced an almost desperate feeling of wanting to watch the documentary. The movie introduced me to two more extraordinary, visionary men, Dr. Peter Fraser, author of *Decoding the Human Body-Field*, and Harry Massey, writer and producer of *The Living Matrix*. From that point on, another shift happened in my life. I soared higher to another level of understanding and awareness as I was introduced to awesome new technologies that could scan and read information in a person's body field. How sweet it was and is!

As an energy healer, I already knew that every living thing is surrounded by energy. And I knew that everyone generates his or her own "body field" of energy. But what I did not know is that researchers had discovered that this body-field acts as a control system, managing the self-healing power of the body. When energy is low, blocked, or disrupted, biology and biochemistry can break down, causing the body's own self-healing power to lapse.

Once more, I felt the feeling of hope move through me—hope for a better solution and that a more complete healing experience might be available through the new science of bioenergetics. As I studied, it all made sense to me.

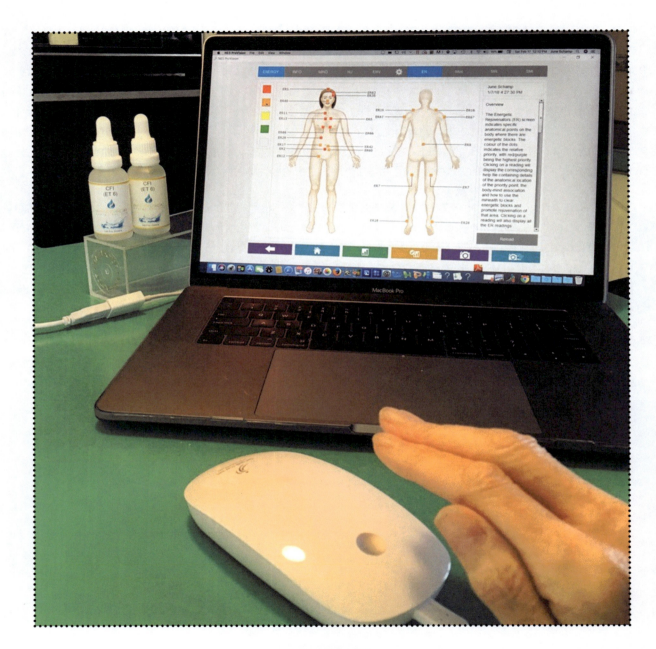

NES Health

During the next eighteen to twenty-four months, I attended classes at NES Health in Tampa, Florida, an international company headquartered in Tampa, Florida with offices in the United Kingdom, and Australia. Founded by Peter Fraser and Harry Massey. Their products and solutions enable health practitioners to radically transform their clients' wellbeing through bioenergetic technology solutions. I submitted the many Client Case Study Reports, completed the tests and all requirements of the NES Total WellNES System, and earned the status of Certified NES Practitioner. Next, I confidently integrated my new wellness system into my energy healing practice. Much love and gratitude to my clients who volunteered their time and patience and helped me complete my studies.

With NES Health knowledge and technology, I can look into my client's energy field and assess information that can lead the client to a more complete healing solution. The NES Total WellNES System is a stunning *new* scientific approach that's restoring energy and health to thousands of people, often when nothing else had worked for them. The NES Total WellNES System offers simple steps that are easy to follow in the comfort of your own home:

- *Assess the Body-Field*. To access the bioenergetic field I use a bio-touch scanner that you attach to your smartphone, tablet, or computer. Place your hand on the scanner and click scan, within minutes you will be able to view your holistic wellness reports.

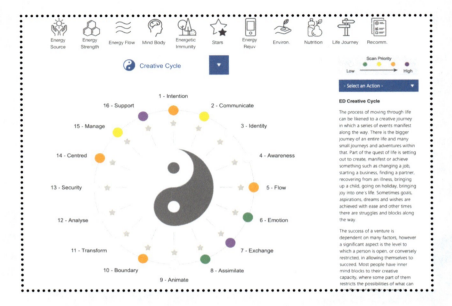

Creative Cycle Chart

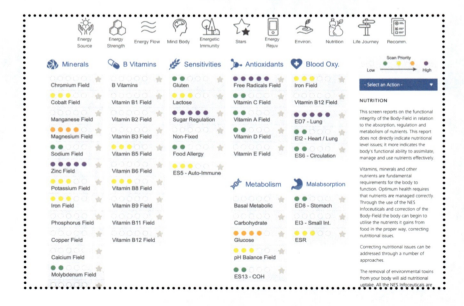

Nutrition Chart

- *Unblock and Rejuvenate*. Your data in the form of various charts and screens will be displayed in your cloud portal after the scan is completed. NES Health's unique miHealth device, with smart bioelectric stimulation, that uses real-time biofeedback can be used to give your body proprietary field correction signals. This can yield a lot of fast results. I also use it to clear away energy blocks and begin to rejuvenate your energy field.

- *Restore Correct Information*. Finally, I provide you with liquid remedies called Infoceuticals. These help to optimize your body-field's energy levels and information flow so that proper communication takes place. A healthy body is all about energy and communication. These remedies have helped thousands of people around the world and they are simple to take by putting some drops into water and drinking the water.

Infoceuticals are information-imprinted water. Drop by drop, the liquid Infoceuticals are encoded with the precise information to correct body-field distortions, restore the body's optimal energy environment, and turn *on* the body's self-repair system so biochemistry functions properly once again! Your cells have receptors to take in not only nutrients but also the information imprinted into the Infoceuticals.

The miHealth is simple to use and, within minutes, releases energy blockages, stimulates trigger points, and brings the body's natural oscillations back to normal. It also assists information delivered by the NES Infoceuticals to flow to where it is needed. It quickly rejuvenates the body's energy field and is excellent after working out or experiencing stress.

TOP 5 "FEEL GOOD" INFOCEUTICALS

Infoceuticals provide the corrective information your human body-field needs to function optimally. The body-field is the master control system that creates and controls the energy your cells need to carry out the trillions of chemical functions they perform every second. With your body-field restored to peak performance your health and wellness is supported and improved.

1. Youth

Youth infoceutical addresses aging of the brain and its lowered ability to produce enzymes and hormones as age increases. Corrects the effects of radiation from the sun and other sources Helps to ease electro-sensitivity for all ages, senility, mental confusion in older people, poor sleep due to melatonin deficiency.

2. Chill

Chill infoceutical encourages a calm mental state. May be helpful hen suffering from constant, long-term stress, especially worry. May support insomnia caused by non-stop thoughts.

3. CFI

CFI inforceutical is for cold and flu immunity. Supports optimal function of tissues affected by colds and flu, supports their health or their return to health. May promote drainage and help re-tune cellular function.

4. Peace

Peace infoceutical supports calm mental state. Enhances the head-heart connection to resolve conflicts between emotions and logical thought as well as memories that have caused disharmony.

5. Energy

Energy infoceutical helps boost energy when you are energetically depleted due to chronic illness, mental exhaustion, stress, toxic exposure, malnutrition or poor breathing.

Empower. Within your cloud portal, informational charts pinpoint where any distortions or blockages exist in your energy field, along with recommendations to repair the problem with Infoceuticals and the miHealth. Also, in the portal are educational videos and a Choice Point Course. Your health is your responsibility, but I do suggest you explore the information and the Choice Point Course. The portal is available for you after your first scan. The information in the portal is awesome and can help you make wiser and more informed choices on your life journey. Your choices will improve through understanding your world better, and you'll learn how to shift limiting mind-body patterns and reduce your stress levels. You'll feel much better—invigorated and with a newfound purpose. All of this reduces entropy; enhances the self-healing powers of the body and mind; and engages an abundance of healthy, vibrant energy for life.

NES Health is the leader in bioenergetics: the study, detection, and correction of energy in living systems. They spent decades mapping out the energy and communication systems of the body. Collectively, these are called the human body-field, which acts as a control system for the body's physical activity.

When this field is underpowered or distorted, it is unable to support the body in an optimal way and the body's cells and systems may begin to fail. Symptoms often begin with simply feeling tired, but they can continue into just about any known health problem. When we improve function of the body-field, and we combine this with good nutrition and lifestyle choices, the body's incredible healing system can take over and begin restoring the body to health.

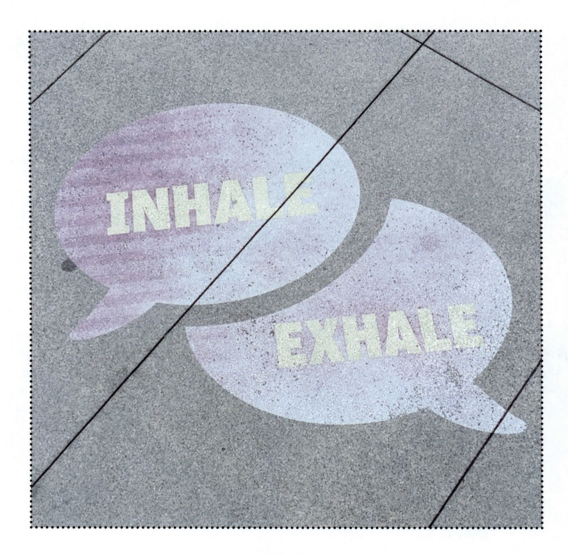

Breathe

Chapter 8

Importance of Managing Our Emotions

As I moved along my personal path of self-growth, many things in my life changed for the better. My life became easier to navigate in the direction I wanted to go. I became more engaged with joyful creativity, along with having more vibrant, healthy energy to complete my tasks. However, in spite of the progress, there were times unwanted emotional reactions would pop up. I would find myself feeling angry, frustrated, anxious, worried, and overwhelmed, especially when I was trying to "do too much," and these feelings would quickly drain my energy. At the time, I really hadn't found a quick, effective way to overcome those negative feelings and shift my mind into a positive, coherent state, which would automatically reverse the entropy that was likely beginning to develop as a result of the negative feelings I was feeling.

At the time, my favorite author was Gregg Braden, author of *The Divine Matrix*, *Human by Design*, *Resilience from the Heart*, *Deep Truth*, and many more books, most of which I have read. He is an extraordinary man, and through his books, he became my mentor.

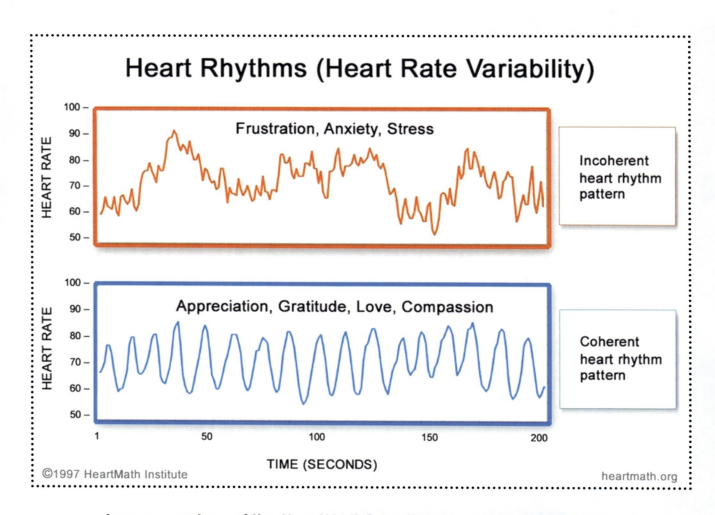

Image courtesy of the HeartMath® Institute – www.heartmath.org.

An opportunity presented itself to me, and I was present at a fabulous gathering, which included Gregg Braden, in the Yucatan, Mexico. We gathered there from December 13 to 22, 2012, to celebrate the end of the Mayan calendar. The event was titled "MAYA 2012: Transform at the Source." The event was magical and transforming, and I was honored to be present with so many awesome "like-minded people" and speakers.

During Gregg's presentation, he demonstrated a scientifically validated stress management technique using his computer and new technology from HeartMath® Institute.* He performed a breathing technique that synchronized his heart rhythms with his breathing while he focused on positive emotions that reduces negative effects of stress, improves relaxation, and builds resilience with just a few minutes of daily use. We saw in real time the reaction of his heart rhythms; his computer screen showed a coherent wave while he focused on his heart as he breathed in a positive attitude of *appreciation*. Similarly, when he focused on a negative emotion of *anger* as he breathed, his heart rhythms produced a chaotic wave. Amazing! See the chart on Page 50.

After I returned from Mexico, I purchased HeartMath technology and practiced the breathing techniques every day. About two weeks later, I became aware of my ability to manage my emotions more easily and quickly noticed my emotional stamina had increased. I went on to complete training and all HeartMath requirements and became licensed as a HeartMath coach/mentor. My favorite technology from HeartMath is the Inner Balance™ trainer. It analyzes and displays our heart rhythm, measured by Heart Rate Variability (HRV), which indicates how emotional states are affecting our nervous system. It is comprised of an application and a clip-on the ear sensor.

* *HeartMath is a registered trademark of Quantum, Inc.*
Inner Balance is a registered trademark of Quantum, Inc.

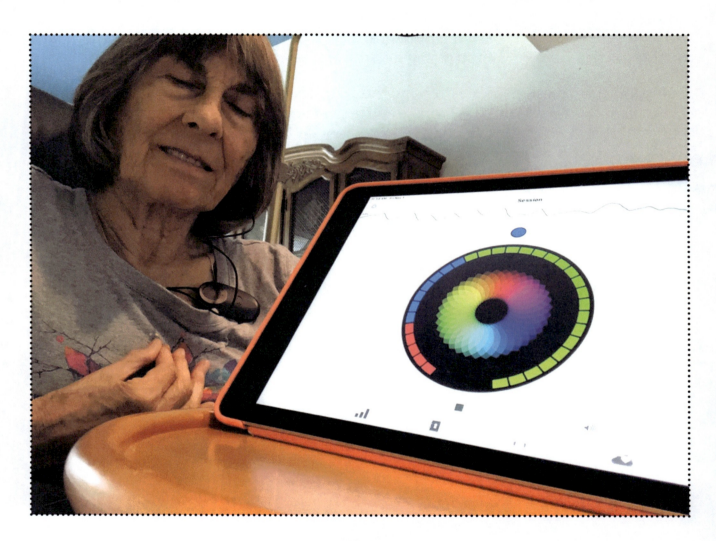

Relax

Bluetooth is available. This simple-to-use technology takes a pulse reading from the earlobe and translates the information from your heart rhythms into graphics on your iOS device or computer. No other technology on the market today tracks your heart rate variability coherence at the refined level of the Inner Balance application and sensor. Also included in the application are options for you to receive immediate training and education, with HeartCloud, (an online platform for all HeartMath devices). This platform gives you the ability to build your training experience, store session data in one location, achieve rewards, celebrate, share your results and see how others in the community are doing. HeartCloud can be accessed anytime from any iOS device or computer.

Synchronizing your breathing with your heart rhythms while focusing on positive, renewing emotions have been shown to reduce negative effects of stress, increase the ability to be calm and build resilience with just a few minutes of daily use. More benefits:

- Neutralize stressful reactions that erode health and composure

- Reduce fatigue and exhaustion

- Improve mental focus under pressure

- Quickly shift from reactive states to calm and balanced states

- Learn to quiet the mind and still restless thoughts

- Builds resilience and faster recovery from stress

- Improves coordination and reactions times in sports

TOP 5 REASONS TO MANAGE EMOTIONS

1. Healthier Brain

Managing emotions is healthy. Suppressing emotions can be unhealthy and lead to brain fog, which is the inability to have a sharp memory or lack of sharp focus. Extreme stress can cause brain fog.

2. Life Control

Emotions are powerful. Your mood determines how you interact with people, how much money you spend, how you deal with challenges and how you spend your time. The more skilled you become managing your emotions the better, clearer, and wiser your decisions.

3. Self-Esteem

Process of learning how to manage your emotions demonstrates how negative thoughts, beliefs and feelings can be recognized, changed and lifted into a positive state.

As the skill is mastered, self-esteem improves.

4. Physical Health

Research shows that emotional distress makes you more vulnerable to physical illness by impacting your immune system. Having good emotional health is a fundamental aspect of fostering resilience, self-awareness and overall contentment.

5. Curiosity

Unchecked emotions often lead us to a state of confusion, uncertainty and fear. One of the great barriers to curiosity is fear. When faced with uncertainty or risk, it seems easier to stay with what is deemed to be safe. New research finds the ability to recognize and manage feelings is beneficial to the creative process. Creativity can calm, heal, and help us live our lives more fully and joyfully.

This valuable tool can help you get your heart, mind, and emotions in sync; improve well-being and performance; and reverse entropy. Engaging our heart's intelligence expands our intuition, and the more connected we become with our heart energy, the more of our heart's intuition is available to us. Amazing scientific information about the energy fields of our hearts is shown in this eBook *The Energetic Heart*: *Bioelectromagnetic Interactions Within and Between People* by Rollin McCraty, Ph.D. HeartMath Institute Research Center (https://www.heartmath.org/assets/uploads/2015/01/energetic-heart.pdf).

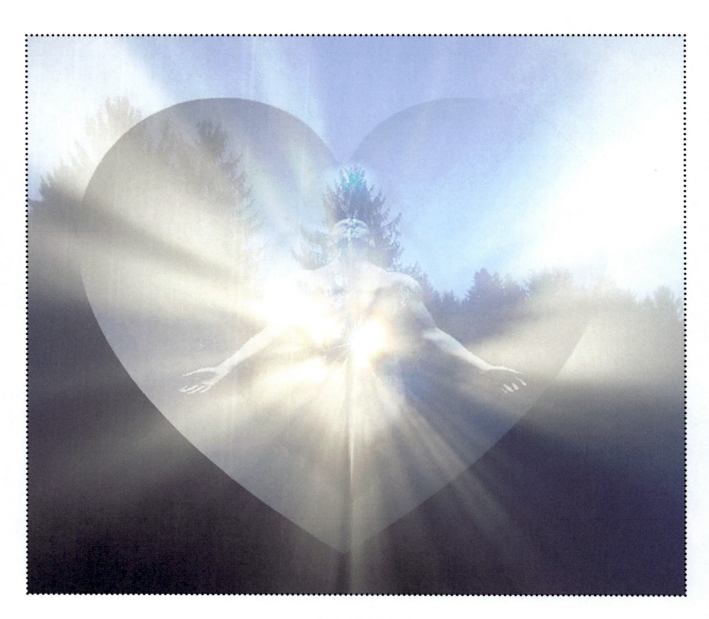

Connection

Part III

BRINGING IT ALL TOGETHER WITH THE FOUR BEAUTIFUL TRUTHS

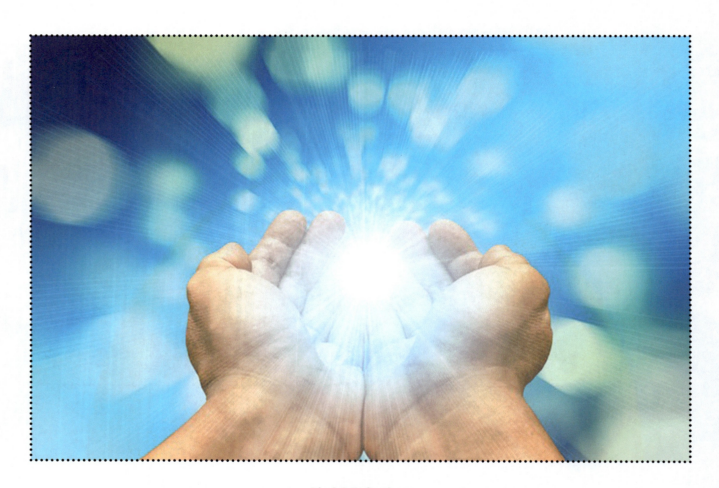

Light Infusion

Chapter 9

Sacred Energy Infusion

In Part I, a map or a guide was developed to give you a basic outline, mostly physical, of what you need to do to begin your journey to longevity with healthy, vibrant energy for life.

In Part II, three extraordinary, revolutionary quantum tools were shared with you to jump-start and supercharge your ability to journey toward longevity with healthy, vibrant energy for life.

In Part III, as you read this section you will receive a sacred energy infusion, an energy that resides between the words and behind the words written in this section of this book. Pay attention and notice how relaxed you are feeling. This sacred energy infusion is an essence or energetic glue that divinely embraces all that is written here. This energy blends with your higher vibrational desires for longevity with healthy, vibrant energy for life and with your committed intention to make it happen. It is the essence that bridges time and space, recodes unhealthy belief systems, and can produces miracles.

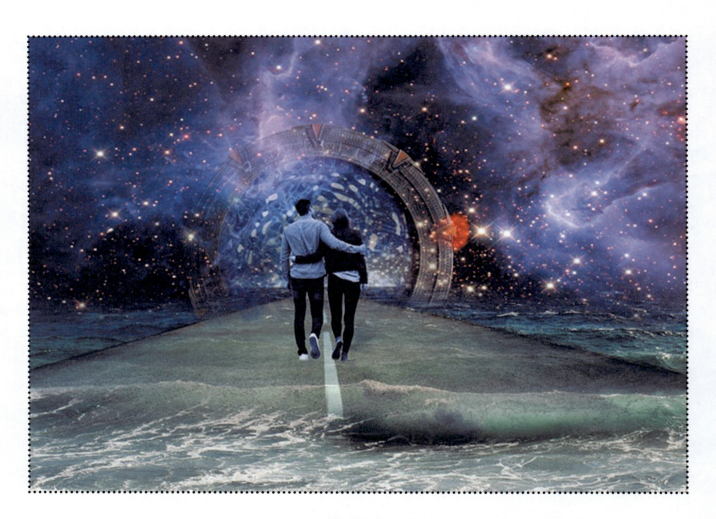

Stargate

Sometime during the mid-1980s I wandered into a metaphysical shop, and a poster on the wall immediately grabbed my attention. I felt blissful peace and love ripple through me. I was captivated and anchored in the space in front of the poster. I noticed a telephone number listed in small print on the bottom of the poster and found myself writing it down and placing the small piece of paper in a secured place in my purse.

The next day, I called the telephone number and became connected to a very special being known as Lazaris. Lazaris is a nonphysical entity, a spark of love and light, channeled through an extraordinary man, Jach Pursel, since 1974. Lazaris is a spark of consciousness that does not have form. For more information about Lazaris and how to access streamed recordings and workshops, visit www.lazaris.com.

I have been studying with Lazaris for over three decades, and Lazaris is more than a source of incredible information and techniques and more than just a teacher to me. Lazaris is a dear friend whose wisdom is woven throughout this book and concentrated in Part III. It is here that I share the four beautiful truths that Lazaris shared with me several years ago. These beautiful truths carry the essence, cohesion, and resonance that is at the core of everything else written here so that living a life of longevity with healthy, vibrant energy for life can become a reality—your reality!

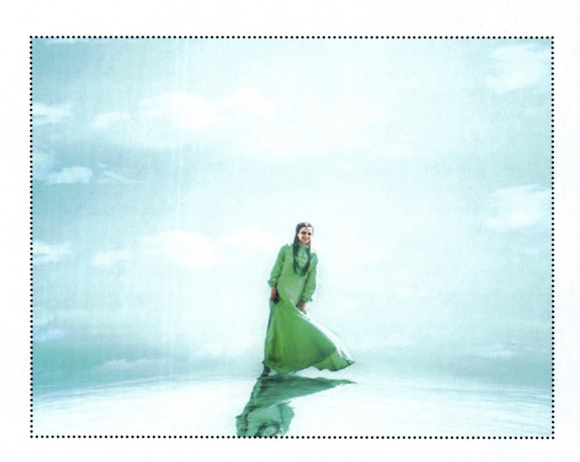

Edge-of-the-world

Chapter 10

The Four Beautiful Truths

The four beautiful truths are the foundation for longevity, the foundation for well-being and that state of mind, and the foundation for being well. The system rests on being loved. Without these embedded magical truths, life becomes a hollow system of demands, expectation, and hard work. With them, it becomes a living matrix for living your life in a state of well-being and in a state of being well.

Truth #1 is that you are *loved*. It is the truth of being loved. Most of you are aware that you are loved and are being loved and you feel you are loved. Most of you are aware and you do understand, and some of you really know it. All of you are aware of it. All of you understand it. But not all really know it yet. So, when you *are* aware of it, you have the information. You know you are loved. And from time to time, you really know it. Sometimes, you forget it. And at times, you act as if you are not aware of it and feel like nobody loves you and longingly want to be loved.

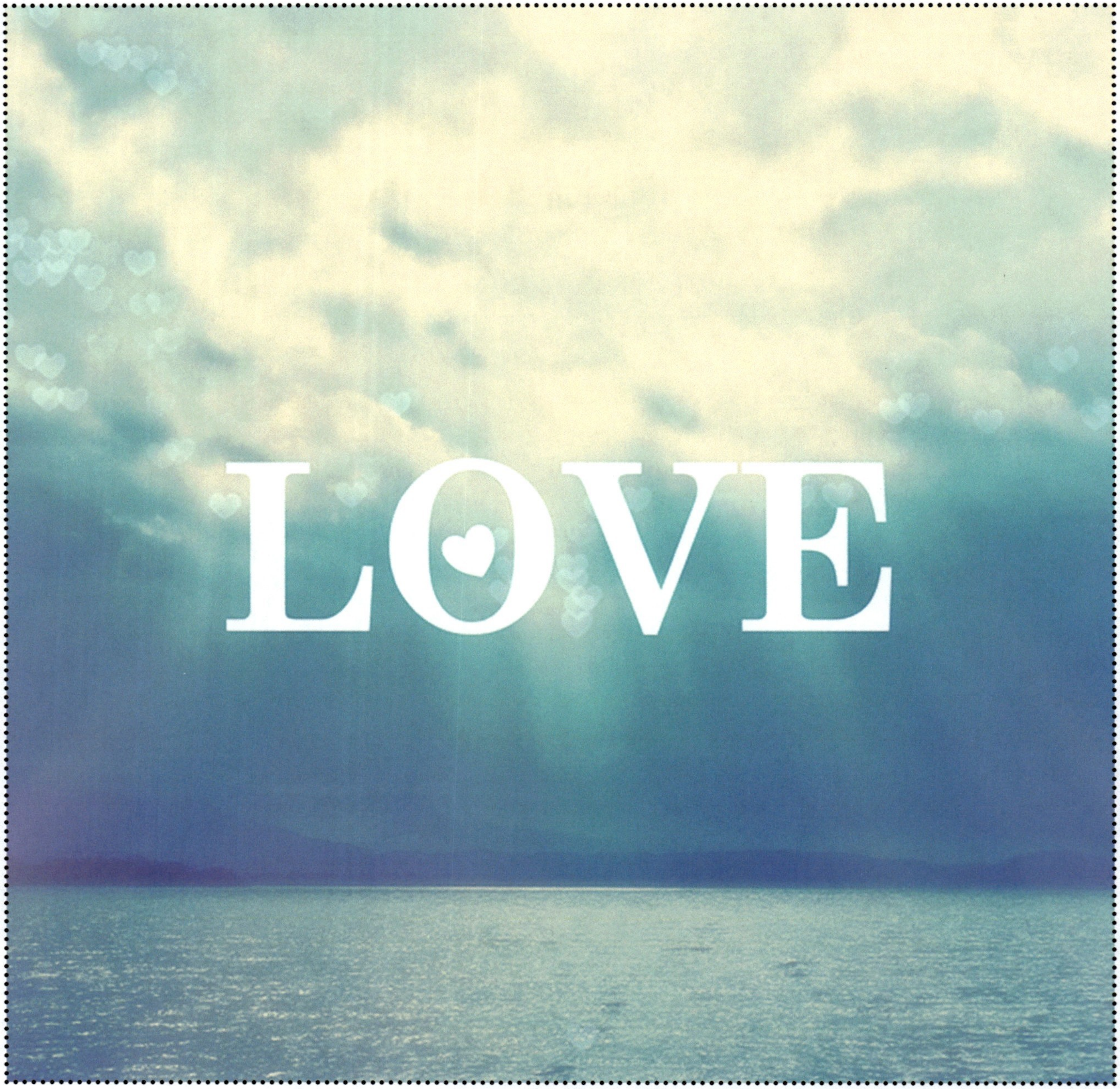
LOVE

So, you lean on it at times, and you count on it, and you use it, but you do not live it. The difference is that you need to remind yourself at times that you are loved. *I am loved.*

It could be helpful to use being loved as a technique. This is the difference between living it and knowing it—where it is automatic, part of the involuntary system; where it just happens like the beating of your heart, like breathing in and out; and where you do not have to remind yourself to do it. You just know it. It just happens. Your body does it instinctively and lets you know that you are being loved.

Being loved is not just this or that. It is a bottomless flow of energy, and there are varying depths to it. We as human beings do not have the ability to know just how deeply and completely we are loved. We don't have measurement and observing devices to completely comprehend the extent and the reach of being loved as we are. It is a truth—a beautiful truth filled with joy and peace, exhilaration and serenity. And it's one of the four beautiful truths that is critical for longevity and to activating this matrix of magic to produce the well-being and all that is being well and all that it can be.

Truth #2 is about *honor*—honoring life and honoring yourself. There are components of honor and of a person who is honorable. Honorable people have qualities about them that are as different as their bodies may be and as different and unique as they may be.

- They have presence and voice.

- They express love, being loved, and being loving.

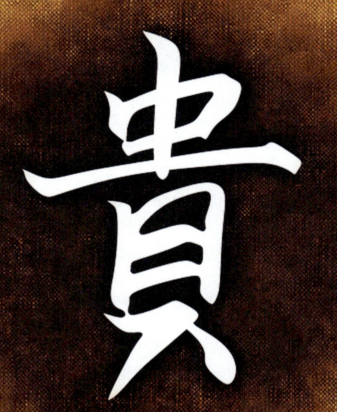

HONOR

- They have gratitude. They express and show gratitude without having to say it. They live it. They are a voice of gratitude.

- They have hope, and that hope is filled with light. A glow is present with their level of hope—not every moment, not every day, but they inspire.

- They are an inspiration.

- They are graciously generous. Generosity comes naturally to them. They do not have to think about it. They just are.

- They have a nobility of soul about them.

To honor life is to experience presence that is in life and to sense that is the voice of life—your life. It's the voice of the love, the gratitude, and the hope that your life holds; the inspiration, the generousness, and the nobility. To honor life, as in your life, is to give attention to these qualities. It isn't all that you experience or see. But do give attention to these qualities, to these energies that you experience in your life and in yourself. Be conscious of your presence and of your voice, of your love and gratitude, and of the glow of light of your hope and the inspiration that you are. Be conscious of your generosity and of your nobility.

This is not all that you are, and these qualities of your being are not the only qualities of your being. But do give attention to these qualities. The key to honoring is to acknowledge and respect—to acknowledge and to then to look back at and see. To respect is to be changed by that acknowledgement; respect the change, no matter how subtle it is. Be aware that you are changed. As you honor yourself and your life, you become an artist at living your life. Develop mastery at living life.

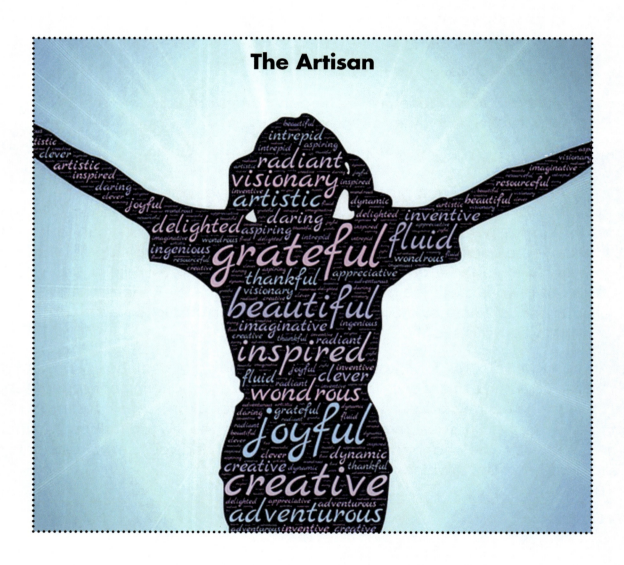

The Artisan

Truth #3 is to be an artist, an artisan of living your life. You practice. You stumble along in the beginning, making mistakes. But you continue to practice, to develop the craft and a certain sense of mastery of life. All those who have mastered an art in sports and creative endeavors have something in common. They all have:

- A sense of discipline, a positive discipline.

- Conviction—a discipline of conviction, and they also have a conviction to their discipline.

- The ability to work clearly, with concentrated intensity of focus and an intensity of concentration. They look more closely with focus in the moment in their element. They are patient as they look more deeply and listen more intently.

- Humility—they are willing to look at everything as if it's brand new, each thing as if it is the first time they are seeing it. They don't assume. They are patient with their humility and humble with their patience. And they practice. They practice their discipline, their conviction, their concentration, their humility, and their patience—and so live life. That is to say they live it fully, both dimensionally and emotionally, just for the thrill of it and allow wisdom to blossom. Practice your art of living life. Be an artisan of living your life. Honor life.

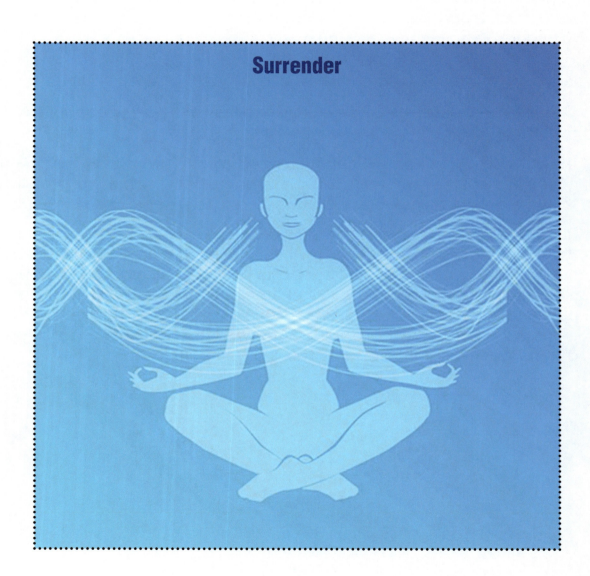

These three beautiful truths form the foundation. Let yourself be loved, honor life, and become an artisan of life. This foundation brings the matrix of longevity, well-being, and being well alive. It is the glue as well as the fuel. I invite you to think about what all of these qualities mean to you in living your life. What does it mean to you to honor life?

Truth #4 is surrender. There is a divine dance of oneness, a celebration of oneness. And it's about recognizing that energy of surrender and surrendering to the moment. It's about letting go of time and space. It's letting go of all expectations and surrendering to whatever the moment may hold. It's about surrendering to the unfathomable, surrendering to that which you cannot fathom. It can be difficult for most people because they need to know where they want to go.

At certain times, of course, you need to know these things. But at certain times, you need to surrender to the uncertainty—to know your boundaries. And yet, there are times to surrender your sense of separateness and be one with all that is.

This fourth truth pulls the other three beautiful truths together. In such a moment when you have surrendered to the unfathomable and to the sense of separateness, you will experience fulfillment. In such a moment, you can be touched by fulfillment. It is not something you can grasp or touch. It is an ideal you cannot reach. In such a moment, you can be touched by fulfillment, creating a whole that is greater than the sum of its parts. You can surrender your sense of your separateness and become part of oneness—a resonance.

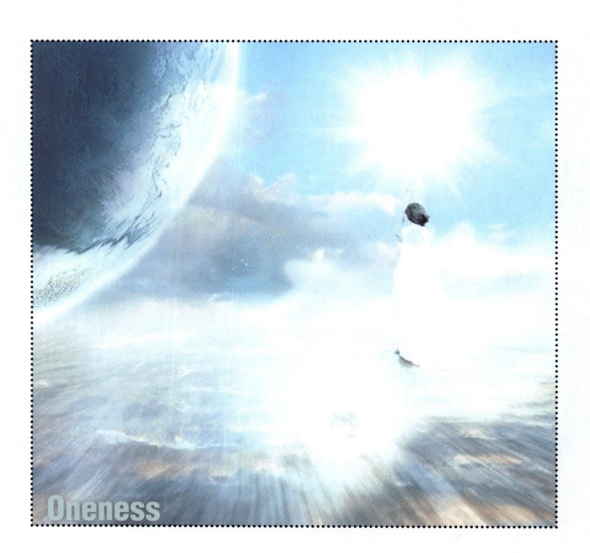

Resonance is the source of all creation in the universe, the force that can turn words into action and desires into reality and with which we attain true dominion. More and more, it is resonance and the future that will determine our reality, not logic and the past.

Note: Each image in this book is imprinted with healing light codes that sync all levels of your being with God/Goddess/All That Is energy. Each image is a powerful portal of light that encourages you to meditate with it or just sit with it in the moment or pause with it as you journey through this book. Become quiet with an image and note how you are feeling, just be an observer of your feelings. Note any intuitive messages that show up—write them down in the white space on most pages.

The images are powerful in helping you connect with your Spiritual Guides. Divine light codes open your heart center and allows for healing and the expression of divine love and compassion. They also radiate frequencies that can close energy leaks, remove strong energy blockages and assist in the return to balance of those who are overly sensitive to other people's emotions and have been energetically traumatized by negative environments. Spend time with the images. Be open to receive.

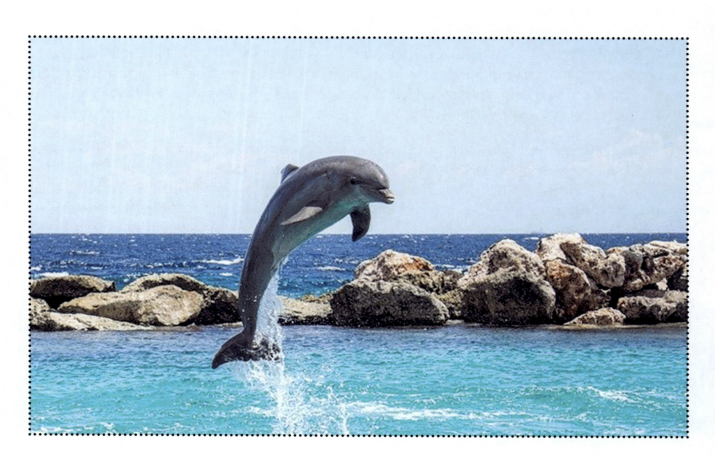

Leap

Conclusion

You are probably at the point of digesting the information written here and deciding if you are ready to take the leap. The human species as a whole has begun an evolutionary leap. Beyond changing, your body systems are evolving, and your brain is beginning to function in a new way with a whole new depth and intensity. Your senses are expanding and evolving. These evolutionary processes, while subtle will become more and more significant and have a greater impact on our lives and on humankind as we live our lives more in the "now" and end our addictions to the past. Importantly, the *resonance* emerging from within these evolutionary changes will make it easier for each of you to create your life the way you want it to be.

With Joy and Inspiration, you and your world can become,
beautifully new and majestic with Love and Light.

—Lazaris

Okay, so you have the map, and you are ready. Take a deep breath and set your intention to journey along the path. Then take a moment to become quiet inside and review the plan:

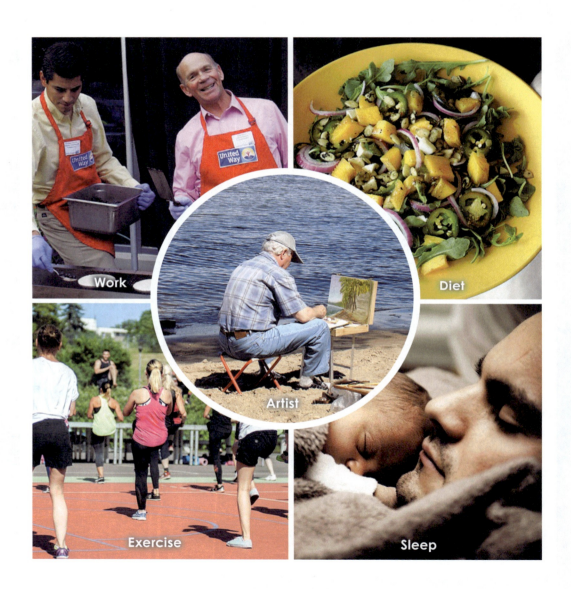

Work

Diet

Artist

Exercise

Sleep

- Upgrade your diet, exercise, and sleep routines. Spend more time outside appreciating the elements. Commit to some kind of work, with or without financial compensation. Make your life richer with lots of playtime. Embellish your work and play with intimacy (as in understanding), caring, and passion.

- If you are ready to travel your path more quickly and achieve your desires sooner, you can reach out to divine revolutionary tools that partner technology, science, and intuition to assist you. *Structured water* acts as a carrier for everything that is life and light-enhancing and repels all that is harmful to your body and mind and creates optimum stamina in your body-mind as you journey your path.

Along the way, issues may surface and you may find yourself confronted with old patterns of feeling "not good enough" or experiencing a lack of confidence to keep going. This suggests an energetic distortion or blockage has surfaced. It is very useful to be able to access the information in your body's energy field that reveals to you the location within, where the unique energetic distortions and blockages are stuck, what may have caused the blockage to form and options for you to correct and restore the energy flow.

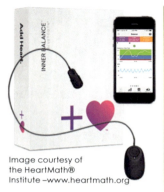

Image courtesy of
the HeartMath®
Institute –www.heartmath.org

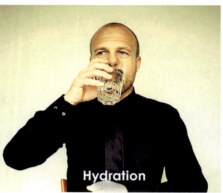

Hydration

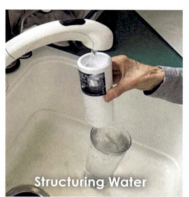

Structuring Water

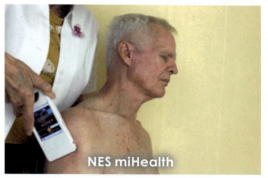

NES miHealth

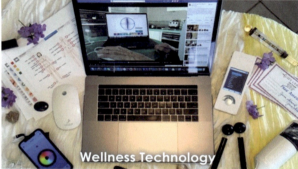

Wellness Technology

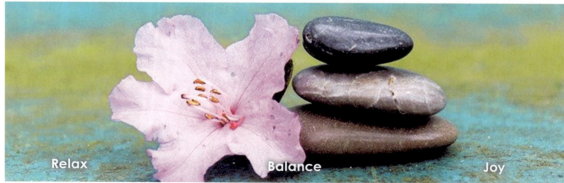

Relax   Balance   Joy

NES Total WelINES System can assess the body-field, unblock and rejuvenate, and restore correct information. This process also changes the template of how your physical body-mind manifests and restores confidence and vitality. In your cloud portal you can view your personal data in the form of charts and reports along with videos, courses, and other educational information to excite you and empower you. As you travel your path toward longevity with healthy, vibrant energy for life, you are likely to become more intensely aware of your humanness, which is a good thing. However, a human being is accompanied with a large array of emotional feelings, which sometimes "show up" at inappropriate times and express themselves in ways we did not intend. These feelings and emotions range from blissful joy and appreciation that enhance optimal health to anger, frustration, and fear that rapidly create an environment of entropy in body and mind.

HeartMath tools and techniques are very appreciated and helpful when "negative" feelings have become unmanageable in the moment. The tools can restore coherence quickly and easily and shift you into an energized and comfortable state of readiness to move forward on your path again.

Become observant of your developing intuition—the feeling that wells up in your heart area with a sense of knowing. This is an energy that, ultimately, is part of the God / Goddess / All That Is energy that exist everywhere in all life. We are one with those loving energies.

It is your sincere intention that invites and activates the energies of the four beautiful truths to wrap around and flow between and around your desire to upgrade your diet, your exercise and sleep routines, and everything you do. They bring miracles and magic and often show themselves to you through your intuition.

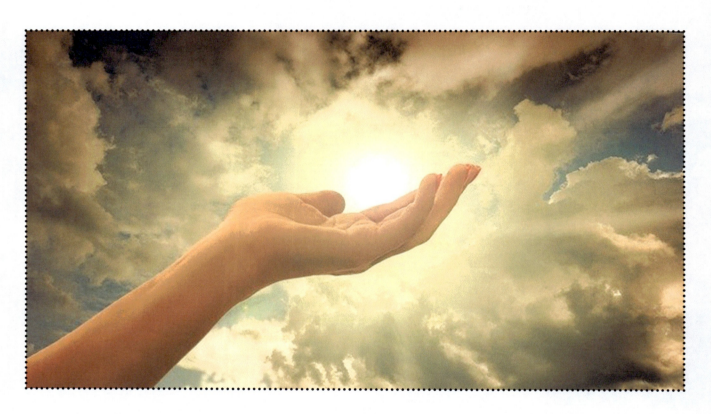

Receive

Trust the flow and get out of your own way. Stop monitoring yourself for signs of change because the mind tools you use for measuring are made up of old thought dialogues, distorted beliefs, and damaged mind-set loops that are no longer accurate and no longer work.

We are all lifting into a new *octave of receivership*, where different, revolutionary tools can help support and lift us. Your unseen friends are with you every day and are there for you to lean on.

Cultivate an inner state of *receivership*. The following mantra can help you begin that process. Speak the following words to yourself, quietly inward or loudly outward. Speak the mantra's verses in sets of three. Speak the set of words a minimum of once daily up to five times per day for best results (five times three equals the mantra being spoken fifteen times):

> I am in the Grace of Receivership
> with the Four Beautiful Truths.
> I am in the Grace of Receivership
> with Truth that I am Loved
> I am in the Grace of Receivership
> with Honoring Myself and Life.
> I am in the Grace of Receivership
> with the Artisan in my Life.
>
> I am in the Grace of Receivership
> with the Resonance of Surrender,
> the Force that turns desires into Reality.
> Thank you God. Thank you God.
> Thank you God!

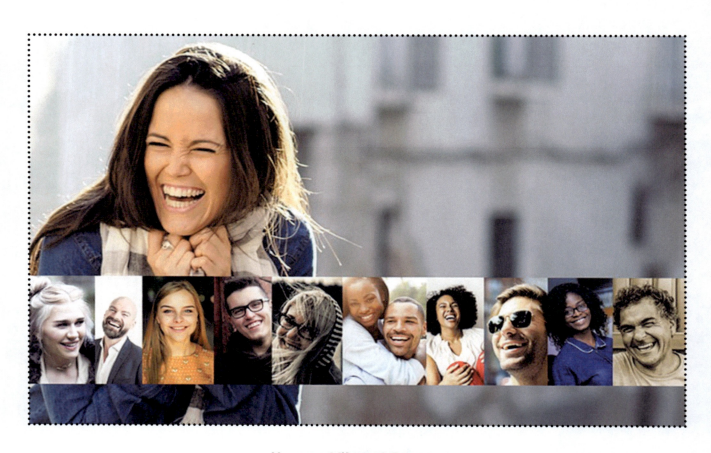

Happy, Vibrant Energy

***

I am here to help you also. I offer a variety of unique coaching sessions that can address any issues you may struggle with as you journey along your path, meeting stubborn energies of entropy. The packages are listed on my website, www.myheartwithin.com, on the Energy Wellness page, the Water Wellness page, and the Emotional Wellness page.

I am in the Grace of Receivership
with Optimal Health,
Wellbeing and an Abundance of All
that is Good for Me.
Thank you God. Thank you God.
Thank you God!

You can adjust the words of these mantras to more useful words that work with your desires in the moment.

Now begin your journey. Upgrade your diet. An easy and simple way is to spray/mist all of your food, cooked and uncooked with structured water.

I am in the Grace of Receivership
with every Cell in my Body
having Healthy, Youthful Beauty
and Vitality.
Thank you God. Thank you God
Thank you God!

May the force be with you.

Namaste!

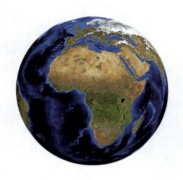

Much love and gratitude to all of my readers and to:

- Lazaris, Jach Pursel, Concept-Synergy www.lazaris.com

- Peter Fraser, Harry Massey, NES Health, www.neshealth.com

- Clayton Nolte, Natural Action Technologies, www.divinewatershop.com

- Doc Childre, www.heartmath.com

- Gregg Braden for showing me the way to HeartMath, www.greggbraden.com

- Barbara Brennan, BBSH, www.barbarabrennan.com

- Dr. Masaru Emoto, https://hado.com/ihm/

To all of my teachers and mentors who have coached and mentored me and will coach and mentor me on my own path.

For more information visit my websites at:

www.myheartwithin.com

www.divinewatershop.com

www.energy4life.com/p/juneschamp

Printed in the United States
By Bookmasters